EFFECTIVE GUIDE ON ULCERATIVE COLITIS, CROHN'S DISEASE AND COOKBOOK

Healthy and delicious recipes with 14 days meal plan for ulcer for both adults and children

Table of Contents

ULCERATIVE COLITIS AND CROHN'S DISEASE (ULCER)

Ulcerative colitis UC: is a known disease which is traced down to persistent swelling of the inside layer of the colon in the digestive system. The inflammation can cause the lining tissue to rupture down, resulting to ulcerations causing bleeding of the colon, which is simply known as ulcer. Inflammation can occupy the whole colon or merely parts of it. Fortunately, ulcerative colitis is treatable. There are certain bacteria found in the colon; they do not cause disorder in the body. However, certain infections result to virus or parasite which enters the colon and eventually cause ulcerative colitis.

Common bacteria resulting to ulcerative colitis are;

- Shigella
- Salmonella
- Campylobacter
- E. Coli

Symptoms

Abdominal Pains

The major symptoms caused by ulcerative colitis include; abdominal pain and diarrhea which consist strains of blood. The signs differ in brutality from mild to stern.

Loss of Weight

The persistent swelling of ulcerative colitis, when not treated, has full effects on nourishment; loss of appetite, weight loss, and stunted growth are common in both children and adults.

Other symptoms

These signs are complications, which are not directly caused by the inflammation in the colon. These complications are general symptoms and signs of soreness and they include;

- Weakness
- Fever
- Bloody stool
- Anemia caused by constant intestinal bleeding
- Nausea
- Arthritis
- Skin sores etc.

Types of ulcerative colitis

Ulcerative colitis is classified according to the location in the digestive system, namely;

Ulcerative proctitis: Inflammation is limited to the area closest to the anus, the only symptom of this disease is rectal bleeding.

Left-sided colitis: this infection extends from the rectum to the sigmoid colon and descending colon. Signs and symptoms are bloody diarrhea, abdominal cramps and ache on the left side, and unexpected urge to use the toilet.

Protosigmoiditis: inflammation affects the rectum and sigmoid colon-the lower end of the colon. The signs and symptoms are bloody diarrhea, abdominal cramps and pain, and the inability to move the intestines despite the willingness to do so.

Pancolitis: This type of infection often affects the entire colon. It causes bouts of bloody diarrhea that may be severe, abdominal cramps and pains, weakness and sudden loss of weight.

The risk factors of ulcerative colitis

It affects roughly the same number of men and women. Risk factors may include:

Age: This disease usually starts under 30 years of age. However, it can occur at any age, and some people may not develop the disease until they are over 60.

Ethnics: White people have the highest risk of developing the disease, and it can occur in any race. If you are of Ashkenazi Jewish descent, your risk is higher.

Family history: If your close relatives (such as parents, siblings or children) have this disease, you are at higher risk.

The difference between Ulcerative Colitis and Crohn's Disease

Ulcerative colitis is identified with Crohn's sickness; this is another constant provocative fiery illness of the digestive organs. Be that as it may, Crohn's illness, differentiating to ulcerative colitis, isn't irresistible just to the colon. Indeed, it includes the small digestive tract and colon. Once in a while it just focuses on the colon. Another persistent gastrointestinal illness, fractious gut problem, shares with ulcerative colitis stomach agony and the runs as its significant side effects. Nonetheless, the wellspring of peevish entrails disorder is thought to be brokenness of the nerves and muscles of the guts since there is no perceptible irritation.

Individuals who may experience the ill effects of Ulcerative Colitis

This infection happens generally in developed countries of the world, and is more regular in enormous urban areas than in the open country. It is assessed that around one million people in the United State experience ulcerative colitis. These Individuals with ulcerative colitis normally contract the illness between 15 – 25 years; however the disorder may maybe begin whenever. All the more additionally, it is accepted that ulcerative colitis is hereditary since it is more normal among relations of people experiencing ulcerative colitis.

Cause of Ulcerative Colitis remains a mystery

The cause for ulcerative colitis stays puzzling. It is accepted that, ulcerative colitis is related to anomalous immunologic responses of the body to the microorganisms found in the colon. There is no known confirmation that diet can cause of ulcerative colitis.

Ulcerative Colitis can cause colon cancer

People who suffer ulcerative colitis are at higher risk of suffering colon cancer. In order to prevent colon cancer, screening colonoscopy with biopsies are recommended on a regular basis, which in most cases performed annually in order to detect precancerous cells so that the infected colon can be surgically removed before cancer develops, and spread.

Diagnosis for Ulcerative Colitis disease

The most acceptable way of diagnosing ulcerative colitis is by colonoscopy.

Colonoscopy is a medical procedure in which a camera attached to the end of a long bendable tube is inserted through the anus up to the colon and then traverses round the colon. Barium Enema procedure can also be used to diagnose ulcerative colitis. This procedure requires X-rays of a barium-filled colon. Colonoscopy is best and more sensitive; it can identify lower levels of inflammation more than Barium Enema. Through colonoscopy, biopsies obtained to confirm the diagnosis.

Medical treatments and care for Ulcerative Colitis disease

Treatment is essential to keep away from complications. Common trouble is bleeding that can end result to anemia. Severe burning can make the colon to malfunction and swell. If not correctly treated as soon as possible, the colon may also rupture and grow to be a clinical emergency. If remedy isn't successful, surgical operation will be the only option.

Other Complications

Severe skin ulcers may occur. A small number of people with ulcerative colitis suffer from severe liver disease, namely Sclerosing Cholangitis. All of these complications involve irritation of the immune system, similar in the colon. Successful treatment of colitis can improve some of these complications, some may not.

Medications for Ulcerative Colitis disease

Ulcerative colitis treatment aims to reduce inflammation in the colon. The most experienced drug to reduce inflammation is a Aminosalicylate, a drug related to aspirin. If Aminosalicylate is ineffective, use corticosteroids (such as prednisone). The third type of drug used is immunomodulators. Any of these drugs help to lower the immune response and thereby reduces inflammation. It may take several weeks to months for the drug to work its best. Biological agents such as Adalimumab can target proteins produced by the immune system.

Biological therapies for Ulcerative Colitis disease

The latest innovation in the treatment of ulcerative colitis is the so-called biological therapy. Biological therapy is a therapy that uses antibodies against molecules produced by the immune system that cause inflammation. The most experienced biological therapy targets a protein produced by the immune system called tumor necrosis factor. Antibodies must be injected intravenously every few weeks.

Whipworm Therapy

A thrilling remark is that contamination with the pig whipworm can be powerful remedy for ulcerative colitis. Scientists consider that the worms that inhabit the colon adjust the immune reaction and thereby lessen the inflammation. In one study, 43% of sufferers with ulcerative colitis improved after consuming pig whipworm eggs for 12 weeks. The motivation for research on whipworm is treatment comes from the observation that ulcerative colitis is not common in developing countries where intestinal parasites are common.

Surgery for Ulcerative Colitis disease

Despite drug therapy, about one-third of patients with ulcerative colitis will require surgery to treat inflammation, prevent or treat cancer, or treat complications such as colon rupture. Surgery to remove the entire colon can cure the person's ulcerative colitis. In the past, they only had an ileostomy (an external bag into which the small intestine was poured). However, surgical techniques have been developed which now encourage the removal of the colon without the need for an ileostomy.

ULCERATIVE COLITIS IN CHILDREN

Children with uncontrolled ulcerative colitis usually grow at a slower rate than normal people, and they may eventually get sick for a shorter time than normal people may. The reason for this is that when active inflammation occurs, appetite is reduced and the amount of food consumed is insufficient. It may be necessary to recommend a high-calorie diet or even supplement nutrition. Children with psychosocial problems due to illness may need a therapist to help them develop strategies to cope with the illness.

Symptoms of ulcerative colitis in children

Ulcerative colitis mostly affects adults, but it can also occur in children. Children with ulcerative colitis may experience a variety of signs of inflammation. These symptoms can vary from mild to severe. Children with ulcerative colitis often experience the peaks and troughs of the disease. They may have been asymptomatic for a while, and then they may experience the onset of more severe symptoms.

Symptoms may include:

- Anemia caused by blood loss
- Diarrhea
- Malnutrition: inability of the colon to absorb nutrients
- Rectal bleeding
- Abdominal pain
- Unexplained weight loss

When ulcerative colitis is very serious, it may cause other symptoms; which may not relate to the gastrointestinal tract. Some examples include:

- fragile bones
- Ophthalmitis
- Arthralgia
- Kidney stones
- Liver disease
- Rashes
- Skin lesions

These side effects make ulcerative colitis hard to diagnose. These symptoms are caused by different underlying diseases, and most importantly, children may have difficulty understanding their symptoms. Teenagers may feel embarrassed and unable to discuss their symptoms.

Diagnosis for kids with ulcerative colitis

There is no perfect test that can be used to diagnose ulcerative colitis in children. However, your specialist can perform different tests to study other symptoms similar to ulcerative colitis.

Extensive tests for ulcerative colitis include:

- Blood tests: (including low red blood cell levels and high white blood cell levels) that may indicate anaemia; a sign of immune system problems.
- The upper or lower endoscope, also called a colonoscopy, used to view the inside of the digestive tract to check for any signs of inflammation.
- A barium enema can help your doctor with better X-ray view of the colon and identify possible areas of stenosis or blockage

Treatments of ulcerative colitis disease in children

The first step is to have a physical examination and record the child's health history. The doctor will ask what made the symptoms worse and how long it took to get better.

Treatment of ulcerative colitis may depend on the severity of the child's symptoms; and how they respond to the disease. Ulcerative colitis in adults is sometimes, treated with a special enema, but children usually cannot tolerate an enema. If they can take the medication, some treatments include:

- Amino Salicylate: reduces inflammation in the colon.
- Corticosteroids: to prevent the immune system from attacking the colon .
- Immunomodulators or TNF-α blockers: to reduce inflammation in the body.

If a child's symptoms do not respond to these treatments and get worse, your doctor may recommend surgery to remove the infected parts of the colon. A child can live without all or part of the colon, although removal will affect their digestion. Ulcerative colitis is likely to reappear in some parts of the colon left after surgery. In rare cases, the doctor may recommend removal of the child's entire colon. Part of the small intestine will be redirected through the abdominal wall so that stool can pass.

Complications in children with ulcerative colitis

In some cases, children with ulcerative colitis require hospitalization, and ulcerative colitis that begins in childhood may also affect most of the colon. The size of the colon is related to the severity of the disease. Suffering from diseases that cause chronic stomach discomfort and diarrhea may make it difficult for children to understand and experience. In addition to physical effects, children will also have anxiety and social problems related to their condition.

Children with IBD may be more likely to encounter the following problems:

- Embarrassing treatment due to their conditions
- Low self-esteem
- Behavioral problems

- Difficulty in formulating coping strategies
- Delays in adolescent development
- Absence from school, which may affect learning

 Children with IBD can also affect family relationships, and parents may worry about the best way to raise their children.

Tips and care for parents and children to cope with ulcerative colitis

- Educate relatives, teachers and close friends about the diseases, nutritional needs and medications.
- Consult any registered dietitian about the diet plan to ensure that your child receives adequate nutrition; seek support groups for patients with inflammatory bowel disease.
- Talk to a counselor when needed.

Reducing flare

Few non-drugs, controllable factors can reduce the symptoms of ulcerative colitis. Reducing stress is very necessary, although it may make symptoms look less severe without actually reducing them. Of course, it is important for patients to take their medications regularly without missing a dose. However, smoking can help to reduce the inflammation of ulcerative colitis, but it is not recommended as a treatment because of its many other harmful effects.

Change of diets is important

Although diet doesn't have an effect on ulcerative colitis, patients are usually advised to eliminate any food found to make symptoms worse. For example, people with

UC may have gastrointestinal symptoms such as bloating, flatulence, and diarrhea that are intolerant to the sugar in milk and lactose. These symptoms may overlap with the symptoms of ulcerative colitis.

Moreover, it is not the cause of ulcerative colitis, reducing milk intake may improve gastrointestinal symptoms in these people. It is important to ensure that the diet is nutritionally adequate, which may require the assistance of a dietitian.

Supplement is ideal

Bleeding because of ulcerative colitis may also cause iron deficiency anemia that is because of the lack of iron garage in purple blood cells within the frame of and those purple blood cells are misplaced to the colon. You may want to complement iron. Drugs used to treat ulcerative colitis can decrease the absorption of vitamins inclusive of folic acid calcium. Supplements such as vitamins and minerals are needed.

Probiotics for People with Ulcerative colitis

Probiotics are made up of bacteria that can give health to the people who consume them. Generally, they are bacteria commonly found in human intestines. Probiotics generally have healthy benefits in several medical conditions. Studies have shown that probiotics can help patients with ulcerative colitis maintain relief. Probiotics have been found in yogurt and some other foods. They have been proven to be effective and sold separately as supplements (but they are not food substances). The effects of probiotics vary widely and depend on the exact bacteria present. Therefore, many probiotics sold may not have beneficial effects. Therefore, it is necessary to carefully select probiotics for treatment based on scientific research.

Drink water always

Chronic diarrhea can lead to dehydration, especially when the individual is unwell and is not eating or drinking too much. It is necessary to maintain sufficient fluid intake. The simplest way to determine if the intake is adequate is to check the amount and color of urine on daily basis. Small or dark urine shows insufficient water intake. The recommended daily amount of water to drink is half an ounce per pound of body weight.

Dealing with UC patient in a relationship

Ulcerative colitis will have a sizable effect on interpersonal relationships, particularly intimate relationships. The ill feeling or desiring to use the toilet often can be socially restricted. These issues may be managed via way of means of right remedy of ulcerative colitis. Medications, which include corticosteroids, can reason temper changes, including melancholy or euphoria. Libido also should be reduced. It could be very vital to reveal those troubles your intimate companion and physician.

Difficulties in travelling

People with relieved ulcerative colitis usually have no problems traveling. If certain symptoms occur, it may be necessary to take some preventive measures, including: asking employees before visiting or using the website to understand the location of the airport and other public buildings, ensuring that changing underwear and wet towels and taking enough medicine as the entire journey continues. If it is necessary to go to a medical institution, please bring a copy of the prescription; it may also be valuable. Discuss your travel plans with your doctor to determine if any other steps should be taken, for example, if your symptoms get worse, you should take other medications for problems.

Food consumption for UC

It is not always easy to know which foods best fuel your body, especially if you have Crohn's disease or ulcerative colitis. Your diet and nutrition is an important part of inflammatory bowel disease (IBD), but no one diet is suitable for everyone. Nutrition not only affects your IBD symptoms, but also your overall health and well-being. Without proper nutrition, the symptoms of Crohn's disease or ulcerative colitis can cause serious complications, including nutritional deficiencies, weight loss, and malnutrition. We provide some tips for healthy eating, which is balanced and nutritious. These techniques are for educational purposes only. You should work with your doctor or a dietitian who specializes in IBD to help you develop a personalized diet plan.

FOOD PREPARATION AND MEAL PLANNING FOR UC (both for adults and children)

Although there is no meal plan for everyone, these tips can help you improve your daily nutrition intake:

- Eat 4 to 6 small food daily.
- Stay hydrated — drink sufficient to hold your urine mild yellow to clear — with water, broth, tomato juice or a rehydration solution.

- Drink slowly and keep away from the use of a straw, which could motive you to ingest air, which may also reason gas.

- Prepare food in advance, and maintain your kitchen stocked with meals which you tolerate well

- Use easy cooking techniques — boil, grill, steam, poach.

- Use a food diary to record your diet and any symptoms you may experience..

How to feed especially when you are in flare

When you have IBD flares, you may need to avoid certain foods, and other foods may help you get the right amount of nutrients, vitamins, and minerals without worsening your symptoms. Your medical team may advise you to abstain from eating and drinking, and you should avoid certain foods to identify foods that cause symptoms. This process will help you identify common foods to avoid during an outbreak. Elimination diet should only be done under the supervision of your medical team and nutritionist to ensure that you are still receiving the necessary nutrients. Some foods may cause cramps, bloating and/or diarrhea. If you have been diagnosed with stenosis, a narrowing of the intestines due to inflammation or scar tissue, or have recently had surgery, you should also avoid many trigger foods. Certain foods are easier to digest and can provide you with the necessary nutrients your body need.

Eating during flare

When you have inflammatory bowel disease (IBD) and are in a flare attack, avoid eating foods that may cause other symptoms, and choose nutritious and nutritious foods. Watch and listen for more information about dietary advice during an outbreak

Feeding when you are recovering

Even after the condition is relieved and the symptoms are reduced or disappeared, it is important to maintain a diverse and nutritious diet. Slowly introduce new food. Remember to keep the water, broth, and tomato juice and rehydration fluid. Please consult your doctor or dietitian before making any changes to your diet.

These foods can help you live healthy and hydrated:

Foods rich in Fiber: Barley, cereals, oat bran, legumes, nuts and whole foods, unless you have an ostomy, intestinal stenosis or the doctor recommends that you continue a low-fiber diet due to stenosis or recent surgery.

Protein: lean meat, fish, eggs, nuts and tofu. **Fruits and vegetables:** Try to eat as much "color" as possible. If they bother you, remove the peel and seeds.

Foods rich in calcium: kale, yogurt, kefir and milk. If you are not lactose tolerant, please choose lactose-free dairy products or use lactase digestive enzymes.

Foods containing probiotics: yogurt, kimchi, miso, sauerkraut.

Foods don't cause ulcerative colitis, but many patients find that eating certain ingredients can exacerbate the condition.

Dietary recommendations for the disease include having frequent small meals instead of large ones and avoiding carbonated beverages, hot spices and high-fiber foods.

Healthy Recipes for Ulcerative Colitis and Crohn's disease

Are you looking for dishes that will not upset your gastrointestinal tract? If you have ulcerative colitis, which is an inflammatory disease of the large intestine, it is not always easy. Meal planning can be a difficult chore for women with ulcerative colitis. Remember that Food does not cause ulcerative colitis; however, many patients find that consuming certain ingredients can exacerbate this condition. Dietary prescription for the disease include: frequent small meals, avoid carbonated drinks, spicy spices and high-fiber foods.

These are some foods that may exacerbate the patient's symptoms:

- Alcohol
- caffeine
- Milk and dairy products (because many people with UC are also lactose intolerant)
- Whole grain legumes (beans and peas)

- Dried fruits berries or anything with small seeds nuts

- Unprocessed vegetables, such as broccoli and cabbage, corn and mushrooms, may be difficult to digest.

- Food with sulfate (as a preservative)

- fatty meats

- acidic foods such as citrus

- Spicy and hot sauce

- All herbs and spices (in some patients instead of chopped or powdered Spices)

- Products containing sorbitol and other sugar alcohols that are used to sweeten sugar-free products

HEALTHY RECIPES AND DIETS FOR PATIENT WITH ULCERATIVE COLITIS CROHN'S DISEASE

The food tolerance of patients with ulcerative colitis is different. Elimination of certain diets can help identify problematic foods. The most common culprits are lactose, high-fat and raw fiber foods, these same foods are easily tolerated during remission. It is also important that every meal contains as many vitamins and minerals as possible, because ulcerative colitis affects the absorption of nutrients during digestion. Despite these potential limitations, a healthy diet is important because ulcerative colitis can lead to nutritional deficiencies. You may need to experiment repeatedly to find out whether certain foods increase gastrointestinal discomfort, so how to avoid aggravating ulcerative colitis in the diet while preparing healthy foods.

Try the following recipes, which do not contain dairy products, citrus, grains and other ingredients that may cause symptoms. Items you may be sensitive to are marked as optional. If any other ingredients cause you trouble, please exclude them.

Try the following recipes to make wholesome home-cooked dishes that will not worsen your symptoms.

Service: 1

Simple roast chicken

No reason to make a fuss about complicated techniques to obtain delicious, rich and simple roast chicken, which is the ultimate comfort food.

Preparation time: 2 hours and 20 minutes

Cooking time: 1 to 2 hours

<u>Ingredients</u>:

- 1 small onion, peeled and sliced into thin slices
- 3 cloves of garlic, peeled and sliced into slices
- 1 5 pounds of chicken, guts removed crushed
- 3 sprigs of fresh tarragon (substitution: teaspoon powder)
- 2 tablespoons of extra virgin olive oil, 1 teaspoon kosher salt,

- ½ teaspoon of freshly ground pepper (optional)

<u>Preparation:</u>

1. Preheat the oven to 375°F.

2. Put onion, garlic, tarragon and thyme into the chicken cavity. Tie the legs with kitchen rope together, closing the opening of the cavity. Pull the wings so that the tip overlaps the top of the breast; tie them in place, and wrap the wings and body with rope.

3. Rub the chicken with oil, salt and pepper (if needed). Place on a baking tray with breasts facing down.

4. Roast the chicken for about 25 minutes. Place the breasts face up and continue

to bake. Baste occasionally with the pan juice until the thermometer is inserted into the thickest part of the thigh without touching the bones records 175°F per 1 hour.

5. Transfer the roast chicken to cutting board; rest for 10 minutes. Remove the strings before carving.

<u>Roasting techniques</u>:

- Very cold meat will not be grilled evenly. Place it on the counter while the oven is preheating. Durable cotton kitchen lines are sold in kitchenware stores most gourmet markets and large supermarkets. Do not use sewing thread or yarn that may contain inedible dyes or unpleasant chemicals.

- Heavy-duty, high-side bakeware is essential to evenly conduct heat. Never replace the cookie table. When baking, the internal temperature of the oven will increase by about 10 degrees. Natural juices will also be re-incorporated into the fiber of the meat, the skin or crusty will dry out a bit to make the dinner more toothy and fleshy.

<u>Nutritional value per meal:</u>

- 180 calories
- 21 grams of protein
- Per 3-ounce serving (without skin)
- 9 grams of fat (2 gram saturated fat)
- 60 milligrams of cholesterol
- 1 gram of carbohydrate

- 0 gram of fiber

- 300 milligrams of sodium

- 217 milligrams of potassium

<u>Nutritional Bonus</u>:

- selenium (30% daily value)

Service 2:

Oven-Poached Salmon Fillets

Baking salmon fillets can produce a moisturizing effect as long as you remember the two basic rules of fish cooking: choose only the freshest Fish, don't overcook it. If needed, sprinkle your favorite sauce on top.

Preparation time: 10 minutes

Cook time: 15 to 25 minutes

<u>Ingredients</u>:

- 1 pound salmon fillet, cut into 4 portions, peeled,

- 2 tablespoons of dry white wine if needed (substitute: broth).

- ½ teaspoon of salt and fresh pepper to taste (optional)

- 2 tablespoons chopped green onions, (1 medium)

<u>Preparation:</u>

1. Preheat the oven to 425°F. Apply cooking spray

2. On a 9-inch glass bakeware or an 8-inch glass bakeware. Place the skinless side of the salmon in the prepared pan.

3. Sprinkle with wine or broth. Season with salt and pepper (if needed), then sprinkle with shallots.

4. Cover with foil and bake until the center salmon is opaque, then start to peel, for 15 to 25 minutes, depending on the thickness.

5. After the salmon is ready, transfer to the plate. Remove all the liquid remaining in the salmon pot.

<u>Nutritional value per meal:</u>

- 246 calories

- 15 grams of fat (3 g saturated food)

- 62 milligrams of cholesterol

- 1 gram of carbohydrate

- 23 grams of protein

- 113 milligrams of sodium

- 434 milligrams of potassium

Service 3:

Salmon chowder

Salmon chowder flavor can makes the meal delicious by adding dill or tarragon. Each herb can give the soup a unique flavor.

Preparation time: 30 minutes

Cooking time: 30 minutes

<u>Ingredients</u>:

- 1 tablespoon of canola oil
- 1 cup of chopped carrots
- 1 chopped celery cup (optional)
- 4 cups of low-sodium chicken broth (check the ingredients on the label)
- 1½ cups of water
- 1 ounce of 12 ounces of peeled salmon fillet, preferably caught in the wild.
- 2 cups of frozen cauliflower florets, thawed and chopped (optional)

- 3 tablespoons of chopped fresh chives or spring onions (substitute: teaspoon Onion powder)

- 1 cup of instant mashed potatoes.

- 2 teaspoons of dried tarragon (substitute: to 1 teaspoon of powder)

- 1 tablespoon of Dijon mustard (optional).

- ½ teaspoon of salt

- Freshly ground pepper to taste (optional)

Preparation:

1. Heat oil in a large pot or Dutch oven over medium heat. Add carrots and celery (if needed) and cook, stirring often, until the

vegetables start to turn brown for 3-4 minutes.

2. Add the broth, water, salmon, broccoli (if needed) and chives or spring onions, then simmer on low heat.

3. Cover the pot and cook, keeping it mild, until the salmon is cooked for 5-8 minutes. Move the salmon to a clean cutting board. Use a fork to peel it into bite-sized pieces.

4. Stir the potato chips (or remaining mashed potatoes), dill or tarragon and mustard sauce (if needed) into the soup until well combined.

5. Add salmon and reheat. Season with salt and pepper (if needed).

<u>Nutritional value per meal:</u>

- 116 calories
- 6 grams of fat
- 26 grams of cholesterol
- 5 grams of carbohydrates
- 15 grams of protein
- 550 grams of sodium
- 490 grams of potassium

<u>Nutritional Bonus:</u>

- vitamin C (50% daily)
- vitamin A (25% DV)
- source of omega-3s

Service 4

Irish Lamb Stew

Before cooking Irish lamb stew, make sure to trim off all visible fat.

Preparation time: 50 minutes

Cooking time: 40 – 45 minutes

<u>Ingredients</u>:

- 2 pounds of boneless lamb leg, cut into small pieces, cut into 1-inch pieces
- 1½ pound of white potatoes, peeled and cut into 1-inch pieces
- 3 large leeks, only the white part, cut into half, washed and thinly sliced
- 3 large carrots, peeled and cut into 1-inch pieces
- 3 celery sticks, sliced into thin slices (Optional)

- One 14 ounces can of chicken broth (check the ingredients on the label for low sodium content)
- 2 teaspoons of chopped fresh thyme
- 1 teaspoon salt
- 1 teaspoon of freshly ground pepper (optional)
- ¼ cup of packed fresh chopped parsley leaves, (optional)

<u>Preparation:</u>

1. Combine lamb, potatoes, leeks, carrots, celery (if needed), broth, thyme, salt and pepper (if needed) in a 6-quart slow cooker; stir to combine.

2. Cover the lid and cook on low heat until the lamb is tender, about 25 minutes or more.

3. Stir in the parsley before serving (if needed).

<u>Nutritional value per meal:</u>

- 250 calories
- 6 grams of fat
- 55 mg of cholesterol
- 30 grams of carbohydrates
- 5 grams of fiber
- 512 milligrams of sodium
- 844 milligrams of potassium

Service 5

Warm Chicken Sausage & Potato Salad

This warm bistro-style salad is the perfect dish to share with guests at the next dinner party.

Preparation time: 30 minutes

Cooking time: 25 minutes

<u>Ingredients:</u>

- 1 pound small potatoes cut in half

- 1 5-ounce bag of arugula (about 4 cups, lightly packed)) (substitute: spinach)

- 12 ounces of precooked chicken sausage cut crosswise into ½-inch pieces (check ingredients on the label)

- 1 cup of cider vinegar (optional)

- 1 tablespoon of maple syrup (optional)

- 1 tablespoon of whole-grain or Dijon mustard (optional)

- 1 tablespoon of extra virgin olive oil and fresh pepper to taste (optional)

<u>Preparation:</u>

1. 1 inch of water to a boil in a Dutch oven. Put the potatoes in a steamer and cover with steam until they are cooked for about 15 minutes.

2. Transfer to a large bowl and add arugula or spinach; cover with foil to keep warm.

3. Cook the sausage in average heat, stir often, until it turns brown and heat for about 5 minutes, then add the arugula into the potatoes mixture.

4. Remove the pot from the heat and whisk in the vinegar (if needed), maple syrup (if needed) and mustard (if needed), scraping off any brown crumbs.

5. Stir gradually in the oil. Pour the seasoning over the salad until the arugula is wilted.

6. Season with pepper (if needed).

<u>Nutrition values per meal:</u>

250 calories

8 grams of fat (1 g sat, 3 g mono)

55 milligrams of cholesterol

30 grams of carbohydrates

20 grams of protein

2 grams of fiber

480 milligrams of sodium

105 milligrams of potassium

<u>Nutritional Bonus:</u>

- vitamin C (45% value a day)

Service 6

Curried Carrot & Apple

This colorful soup is simple and delicious. Use apples that cook easily and soft. Mackintosh is great.

Preparation time: 1 hour

Cook time: 35 - 45 minutes

Ingredients:

- 1 tablespoon of extra virgin olive oil
- 1 large onion, chopped (2 cups)
- 1 celery stalk, chopped (optional) 1 tablespoon curry powder (substitute: turmeric powder)
- 5 large carrots, peeled and thinly sliced (3 Cup)

- 2 large McIntosh or other apples, peeled and chopped (3 cups)
- 1 bay leaf
- ½ teaspoon of salt
- fresh pepper to taste (optional)
- 1 tablespoon chopped fresh parsley, dill or basil for garnish (optional)

Preparation:

1. Heat oil in a large pot or medium stock pot over medium heat.
2. Stir the onion and celery (if needed); cook until the onion is soft and translucent, for4 –5 minutes; not brown.
3. Add curry powder or turmeric. Then add carrots, apples and bay leaves. Stir

well over medium heat for 2 minutes, and then add broth and salt.

4. Bring the mixture to a boil, by reducing the heat.

5. Cover the pan tightly and simmer for 15 -20 minutes, until the carrots and apples are soft.

6. Take out the bay leaves. Use a tablespoon to transfer the soup solids to a food processor, add about cup of broth; process into a smooth slurry. Pour the puree into the soup.

7. Reheat and season with pepper (if needed). Serve piping hot food and sprinkle each serving with fresh herbs if you want.

<u>Nutritional value per meal:</u>

- 80 calories

- 2 grams of fat (1 g saturated fat, 0 gram of monosaccharide)

- 3 grams of cholesterol

- 10 grams of carbohydrates

- 3 grams of protein

- 3 grams of fiber

- 188 grams of sodium

- 230 grams of potassium

<u>Service 7:</u>

Roasted Asparagus with Caper Dressing

Roasting will thicken the grassy taste of asparagus; caper sauce provides saltiness. Serve with grilled fish or meat.

Preparation: 25 minutes

Cook time: 15 minutes

<u>Ingredients:</u>

- 2 bunches of asparagus (about 2 pounds)
- 1 tablespoon plus 2 teaspoons extra virgin olive oil, separated.
- ¼ teaspoons salt and fresh pepper, separated (optional)
- 2 Cups of chopped scallions, cupped parsley leaves,
- 3 tablespoons of rinsed capers (on-line packaging and salt-packed capers in gourmet stores)
- 2 tablespoons of white wine vinegar (optional)

<u>Preparation:</u>

1. Preheat the oven to 450°F

2. Trim the hard ends of the asparagus; place on a baking sheet.

3. Sprinkle 1 tablespoon of oil, salt and teaspoon pepper (if needed) on the asparagus; toss the coat.

4. Spread out a layer and roast, rotating once halfway, until the asparagus starts to soften and brown (12 to 14 minutes).

5. Transfer to serving plate. At the same time, put the shallots, coriander, capers, vinegar (if needed), the remaining 2 teaspoons of oil and teaspoon of pepper (if needed) into the blender and blend well until the ingredients are chopped or flattened. Serve asparagus with seasoning.

<u>Nutritional value per meal:</u>

- 108 calories

- 5 grams of fat (1 gram of saturated fat)

- 10 grams of carbohydrates

- 7 grams of protein

- 5 grams of fiber

- 346 milligrams of sodium

- 520 milligrams of potassium

<u>Service 7:</u>

Butternut Squash Soup with Lemongrass

Abdominal healing is improved by using this soothing low FODMAP soup. Peeled, cooked and mixed vegetables are easy to digest during ulcerative colitis attacks.

Preparation time: 1 hour

Cook time: 40 – 45 minutes

<u>Ingredients:</u>

- 2 tablespoons of extra virgin olive oil
- 4 of cups peeled and cubed butternut squash
- 2½ cups of chopped carrots (about 3 large carrots)
- 1½ tablespoon of chopped fresh ginger
- 1 tablespoon of lemongrass sauce
- 1 teaspoon of turmeric powder
- ½ tablespoon of kosher salt
- 4 cups of low-sodium vegetable broth.
- ½ cup plus 4 tablespoons of coconut-milk yogurt, separately.
- light green vegetables or fresh basil for garnish (optional)

1. Heat oil in a Dutch oven or large stockpot in a medium heat. Add squash and carrots; cook for 7 minutes, stirring occasionally, until light golden brown.

2. Stir in ginger, lemongrass paste, turmeric and salt; cook for 2 minutes, until fragrant.

3. Add broth and increase heat until the mixture boils. Then reduce the heat to a low level.

4. Cover the pot and cook for about 40 to 45 minutes, until the vegetables are tender.

5. Carefully pour the mixture into the blender; add a cup of yogurt. Remove the central part of the blender cover to allow steam to escape, fix the cover on

the blender. Put a clean towel on the opening of the lid. Processing until smooth.

6. Divide soup evenly into several bowls. Add yogurt into each serving, and garnish with fresh basil or microgreens, (if needed).

<u>Nutritional value per meal:</u>

- 220 calories
- 8 grams of fat (2 gram of saturated fat)
- 35 grams of carbohydrates
- 7 grams of protein
- 6 grams of fiber
- 546 milligrams of sodium
- 745 milligrams of potassium
- 138 grams of calcium

<u>**Service 8**</u>

Fried Rice with Miso-Turmeric Vinaigrette

The fiber content of white rice is lower than brown rice, so when your UC symptoms occur, white rice is easier to digest.

Preparation time: 40 minutes

Cook time: 20 – 25 minutes

<u>Ingredients:</u>

- 2 tablespoons of unseasoned rice vinegar
- 2 teaspoons of sesame oil (unbaked)
- 2 teaspoons of white miso sauce
- 1 teaspoon of salt
- ½ tablespoon of freshly grated ginger
- 2 tablespoons of turmeric powder
- 2 cups vegetable oil
- 2 cups of roughly chopped cabbage Choy
- 1 cup matchstick carrots

- 3 cups cooked white rice
- 2 tablespoons of low-sodium soy sauce
- 3 large eggs, whisked
- 2 tablespoons of eggs
- 2 tablespoons of chopped fresh basil

<u>Preparation:</u>

1. Combine vinegar, sesame oil, mio, ginger and turmeric in a small bowl, prepare the seasoning; stir with whisk. Set aside.

2. Heat the vegetable oil in a large pot to medium high. Add cabbage and carrots; cook for 5 minutes, stirring often, until soft. Add the rice and soy sauce, and then press the rice evenly into the frying pan. Cook for about three minutes until the rice starts to become crispy. Toss and combine.

3. By pushing the rice and vegetables to all sides, a large opening is created in the center of the pot. Pour in the eggs and keep stirring until the eggs are disrupted (about 1 to 2 minutes).

4. Mix the eggs and rice well, and stir in the basil. Place the fried rice evenly between the some plates.
5. Top with drizzle turmeric balsamic vinegar

Nutritional value per meal:

- 319 calories
- 20 grams of fat (4 gram saturated fat)
- 140 milligrams of cholesterol
- 443 milligrams of sodium
- 32 grams of carbohydrates
- 1 gram of fiber
- 9 grams of protein
- 70 milligrams of calcium
- 90 milligrams of potassium

Service 9

Sweet Potato and Lentil Soup

When your UC is in remission, legumes (such as lentils) can provide you with the ideal fiber and protein dosage.

Preparation time: 50 minutes

Cook time: 25 – 40 minutes

Ingredients:

- 2 tablespoons of extra virgin olive oil
- 1 cup of chopped yellow onions
- 3 garlic cloves
- 2 tablespoons of tomato paste
- 2 teaspoons of cumin powder
- 2 tablespoons of Garam masala
- 1 large sweet potato, peeled and cut into thin slices. Fragments (about 2 cups)
- 1 cup uncooked brown lentils
- 4 cups low-sodium vegetable soup
- 2 cups water
- 1 (14.5 ounces) can roast tomatoes
- 1 teaspoon of kosher salt
- 1 bunch of kale, stalks removed and chopped fresh parsley for garnish (optional)

<u>Preparation:</u>

1. Heat the oil to medium in a large saucepan or Dutch oven.
2. Add onions; cook for 5 minutes, until tender. Add garlic, tomato paste, cumin and Garam Masala; cook for 2 minutes, stirring occasionally.
3. Add sweet potatoes; stir and cook for 5 minutes. Add the lentils, add the stock, water, tomatoes and salt; bring the mixture to a boil.
4. Reduce the heat, simmer on low heat, and cover, until the lentils are cooked and the sweet potatoes are tender, about 30 to 35 minutes.
5. Pour in the kale and stir and cook until the kale is wilted for about 2 minutes.
6. 3 Divide evenly into several bowls. You can garnish with fresh parsley (If needed).

Nutritional value per meal:

- 250 calories
- 6 grams fat (1 gram of saturated fat)
- 652 milligrams of sodium

- 19 grams of carbohydrate
- 4g fiber
- 12 grams protein
- 124 milligrams of calcium
- 6 milligrams of iron
- 604 milligrams of potassium

<u>Service 10</u>

Zucchini Noodles with Ginger-Peanut Sauce

This delicious lunch is also low in FODMAP and low carb, which is especially important for UC patients on steroids.

Preparation time: 30 minutes

Cook time: 15 - 20 minutes

<u>Ingredients</u>:

- 3 tablespoons of natural creamy peanut butter
- 2 tablespoons low-sodium soy sauce
- 1½ teaspoon of fresh ginger juice
- 2 teaspoons of lime

- 2 tablespoons of pure extra virgin olive oil, separately
- 1 ounces (14 ounces), drain the firm tofu cubes, drain, pat dry, and cut into 1-inch pieces
- ½ teaspoon of kosher salt
- 1½ cup of matchstick carrots
- 1 red sweet pepper, thinly sliced
- 4 medium zucchini, thinly sliced and spiraled into thin noodles

<u>Preparation:</u>

1. In a small bowl, combine the peanut butter, soy sauce, ginger, lime juice and maple syrup and mix well. Set aside. Heat a tablespoon of olive oil in a nonstick pan.
2. Add tofu; cook until the tofu is golden and crisp, stirring occasionally. Season the tofu with a small spoon. Salt; transfer to a plate.
3. Season with the remaining ¼ teaspoon of salt.
4. Put the zucchini noodles in the pot; cook for 2 to 3 minutes, turning

frequently to heat, but not fully cooked. Add tofu and half of the peanut butter to the frying pan.

5. Place the zucchini noodle mixture evenly between the some plates.
6. Drizzle the remaining peanut butter on top.

<u>Nutritional value per meal:</u>

- 308 calories
- 17 grams of fat
- 3 grams of saturated fat;
- 512 milligrams of sodium
- 18 grams of carbohydrates
- 5 grams of fiber
- 17 grams of protein
- 122 milligrams of calcium
- 675 milligrams of potassium

It's OK to try any of these recipes severally, at any convenient time. They are totally healthy and delicious. The listed ingredients are essential; they will help to heal and improve your ulcerations. You can exclude any of the ingredients if it causes discomfort in your body. Enjoy!

www.ingramcontent.com/pod-product-compliance
Lightning Source LLC
Chambersburg PA
CBHW061728250726
48657CB00002B/821

MAÎTRISEZ L'INDICE GLYCÉMIQUE BAS

UN GUIDE COMPLET POUR UNE ALIMENTATION ÉQUILIBRÉE ET ÉNERGÉTIQUE

AARÂV KAPOOR